101 Delicious

Recipes on Ketogenic Diet

For Quick and Guaranteed Weight Loss and Healthy Living.

Table of Content

Introduction

I want to thank you and congratulate you for downloading the book, *"101 recipes on Ketogenic diet recipes to stay healthy"*.

There are different ways to stay fit and using the Ketogenic way to stay fit is a healthy trend now. In this book, I have shared some basic idea about Ketogenic diet and the benefits that you can derive by following it. it will help you grow your confidence when you follow the diet.

This book contains different ketogenic recipes that can be enjoyed by you while you are on a ketogenic diet. They are divided into different sections, like a recipe for breakfast, lunch, dinner and desserts too! However, there are no hard and fast rules that you should enjoy each item as mentioned in the book.

Cook them when you want and enjoy each recipe. There is a combination of various food items so that you do not feel boredom while you are on a Ketogenic diet. The recipes mentioned here are for different servings and you can alter the ingredients easily depending upon the quantity of food served by you.

You will get almost every ingredient in your nearby shopping mall, however, if you do not get anything there you may always try at online stores. You will get the ingredients easily there. So, enjoy your Ketogenic diet plan and do cook each recipe to enjoy the taste of these low card high fat recipes.

Thanks again for downloading this book, I hope you enjoy it!

Chapter 1

Ketogenic Diet- a step towards wellness

Often termed as Keto, the Ketogenic diet is a high fat, low card diet which converts your body into a fat burning machine. It shares many similarities with other low carb diets like Atkins diet but has a potential health impact.

When you undertake this diet the total carbohydrate intake will reduce replacing that with fat. By reducing the carbs in your body, it falls into a state that is known as ketosis. During ketosis, your body becomes efficient at burning the fat into energy. Apart from that this diet also helps in converting the fat into ketones in the liver that is responsible for supplying energy to the brain.

There are different positive health impacts of this diet plan that includes a reduction in blood sugar and insulin level, weight loss and much more. This diet does need you to count your calories while you lose weight, it is so filling that you feel energized whole day while you follow this diet plan.

1. a Different Types of Ketogenic Diets

The ketogenic diet is helpful in letting you gain power, speed, endurance and muscles. For this, there are different types of ketogenic diet. They are discussed below.

- Standard ketogenic diet (SKD): This is a very low carb, high fat, and moderate protein diet. This diet contains 5% carb, 75% fat and 20% protein. It aims at eating the minimum amount of carbs at any time of the day and is the most popular ketogenic diet.
- Cyclical ketogenic diet (CKD): as the name suggest there is a change in the diet after few alternate days. You consume low carb diet for few days and then there is a period of higher carb feed. It is known as carb-loading.
- Targeted ketogenic diet (TKD): this diet let you eat carbs before some time of your exercises. It mainly refers to carb with Glycemic Index that does not upset stomach easily.
- High-protein ketogenic diet: this is like SKD but it allows one to use more protein. The ratio of fat, carb, and protein here is 60:35:5.

In this book, we well mainly refer to Standard Ketogenic diet as CKD and TKD are advanced methods that are practiced by professional.

1. b. Who should avoid ketogenic diet

Ketogenic Diet is ideal for anybody who wants to stay healthy. It mainly depends upon ketosis. The term 'Ketogenic' has come from the fact that your body during following this diet produces small fuel molecules that are known as 'ketones.' You will know about it in details in next chapter.

This diet is beneficial for almost everybody but few people must avoid this diet. They are

- People who are suffering from Diabetes and is on medication.
- Someone who is breastfeeding must avoid this diet for the time being.
- People who are under medication for being suffering from High Blood pressure must avoid this diet.

Chapter 2

Benefits of Ketogenic Diet

Before you know about the benefits derived from Ketogenic Diet, let's explain how this diet is helping you to lose weight.

As already mentioned in Chapter 1.b that during this diet 'Ketones' are produced. This alternative fuel for your body is used when the glucose or blood sugar is short in supply.

For producing ketones, you need to eat very few carbs, as they break down to blood sugar quickly and moderate amount of protein as if you consume an excess amount of protein it may also be converted into blood sugar.

From fat, the ketones are produced in the liver and then used as fuel throughout your body. Even your brain uses them as the brain is the hungriest organ and it needs to consume a lot of energy every day. It cannot survive of fat directly and thus it needs glucose or ketones.

While you are on a ketogenic diet, your body converts its fuel supply in such manner that it runs entirely on fat. The level of insulin minimizes and the process of fat burning increases. Your fat store is accessed easily and they are burned off. If you want to lose weight this is very effective and apart from that it also provides you with energy.

When your body is producing ketones, it is known as Ketosis and the best way to be in ketosis is fasting. However, it is not possible to fast forever, hence by following the ketogenic diet you can get similar advantages of fasting.

Once you know how ketogenic diet helps you let's go through the benefits of Ketogenic diet

Lose Weight

By following the ketogenic diet, you can lose weight easily. The main reasons are that during this diet your body is converted into a fat burning machine. Thus, while you are enjoying your 'keto' meals you are also stepping forward to lose weight. Your insulin level drops greatly while you follow this diet, hence an ideal circumstance is created where you lose weight without feeling hungry.

Reverses Type 2 Diabetes

The main cause of Type 2 diabetes increases blood sugar level in your body. Your body is unable to control the insulin level and thus suffer from high blood sugar. While you are on the ketogenic diet your insulin, the level is controlled and thus your diabetes is also under control.

Better mental focus

During the process of ketosis, there is a steady flow of ketones to your brain. Apart from that during this diet, you also avoid big swing in your blood sugar level. Hence, there is increased focus and your concentration level improves. A proper keto diet will help you in the reduction of a headache, irritations and the overall concentration will increase over time.

Many people believe that carbs in required for maintaining the mental focus and for the proper functioning of the brain. This is true but when ketones are there, there is no need of carbs. You will feel energized and mentally focused.

Helpful in other health conditions

Research has shown that ketogenic diet is also very helpful in combating different health conditions. They are

- Heart disease: as ketogenic diet helps in improving various risk factors like HDL levels, body fat, blood pressure and blood sugar.
- Cancer: this diet is presently used while treating different types of cancer as it helps in minimizing the growth of the tumor.
- Alzheimer's disease: it is useful in reducing the symptoms of the diseases and slows down its progression.
- Epilepsy: people suffering from epilepsy need to consume less medication if they are on this diet. It is helpful in reducing massive seizures.
- Polycystic Ovary syndrome: with the help of ketogenic diet the insulin level can be reduced. Insulin plays a major role in POS. hence; ketogenic diet is useful for controlling it.
- Acne: you eat less sugar from the processed food and the insulin level is lowered. So, there is an improvement in acne.

Chapter-3

Foods to Eat and to Avoid during Ketogenic diet

Foods to Eat

While you are on a Ketogenic diet you can fill up your refrigerator with the following food items.

Meat: Red meat, ham, steak, sausage, chicken, bacon, and turkey.

Fatty fish: Such as salmon, tuna, trout, and mackerel.

Eggs: Preferable omega-3 or pastured whole eggs.

Butter and cream: Prefer grass-fed when possible.

Cheese: Unprocessed cheese (cheddar, cream, goat, mozzarella or blue).

Nuts and seeds: Pumpkin seeds, Almonds, chia seeds, flaxseeds, walnuts, etc.

Healthy oils: Primarily coconut oil, extra virgin olive oil, and avocado oil.

Avocados: freshly made guacamole or Whole avocados.

Low-carb veggies: Most green veggies, onions, tomatoes, peppers, etc.

Condiments: You can use pepper, salt, and various healthy spices and herbs.

Foods to Avoid

Say No to these food items whenever possible and when in Ketogenic diet simply forget about them.

Any food item with high carbs should be limited totally.

Apart from that reduce or eliminate these food items from your list

Sugary foods: Soda, smoothies, fruit juice, cake, candy, ice cream, etc.

Grains or starches: Wheat-based products, pasta, rice, cereal, etc.

Beans or legumes: Peas, lentils, kidney beans, chickpeas, etc.

Fruit: All fruit, except small portions of berries like cranberries.

Root vegetables and tubers: Potatoes, carrots, sweet potatoes, parsnips, etc.

Low-fat or diet products: they are processed highly and thus often are high on carbs.

Some sauces: as they contain sugar and unhealthy fat.

Unhealthy fat: Limit your intake of processed mayonnaise, vegetable oils, etc.

Alcohol: Due to its carb content, alcoholic beverages are strict no during the Ketogenic diet.

Sugar-free diet foods: These are often high in sugar alcohols and are highly processed. It affects the ketone levels in certain cases.

Bottom Line: Avoid carb-based foods like sugars, legumes, grains, rice, potatoes, juice, candy, and even most fruits.

Chapter 4

Recipes on Ketogenic Diet

Your body relies on either carbohydrates or fat for the energy that helps you run every day. The ketogenic diet or the high fat low carb diet is mainly designed so that your body gets enough fat to convert to ketones that will supply it with the necessary energy. It cut downs the carbs so that carbs do not get accumulated in your body.

As suggested earlier while you are on a Ketogenic diet you can try out the following recipes. I have divided them as per Breakfast, lunch, dinner, snacks and others so that you can enjoy them as per your requirement.

Chapter 4.1

Keto Breakfast recipes

Start your day with healthy Keto breakfast recipes. They are easy to make and tasty to eat. Enjoy them while staying fit.

1. Egg Muffins

Make these hand muffins for either enjoying your breakfast at your home or carrying them along with you.

Ingredients (4 servings)

- 6 eggs
- Finely chopped 1 – 2 scallions
- 4 – 8 thin slices of cooked bacon or salami or air-dried chorizo
- 3½ oz. shredded cheese
- 1 Tbsp. red or green pesto (optional)
- Pepper and salt

Instructions

- Preheat the oven to 175°C or 350°F
- Then Chop bacon and spring onion.
- Mix eggs with pesto and seasoning and whisk it. Gradually add cheese and stir it.
- Add chorizo, bacon, and salami to the muffin form and then place the batter in it.
- Depending upon the size of the muffin, bake the batter for 15 to 20 minutes.
- To make it keto you can add more fat to it. You can add some more butter to make it keto.

2. Spinach, Ham, and Ricotta Casserole

Enjoy the delicious flavor of Ricotta while biting into ham.

Ingredients (4 servings)

- 6 large eggs
- 1/2 cup ricotta cheese
- 1/8 cup heavy whipping cream
- ½ small yellow onion
- ¼ tsp. salt
- ½ Tbsp. Herb and Garlic seasoning
- 4-ounce water squeezed frozen spinach
- 1/4 pound diced ham

Instructions

- Start by chopping yellow onion and in the mean time preheat oven at 350°F
- Blend together 4 eggs, chopped onions, heavy whipping cream and ricotta cheese. Keep aside.
- Take another bowl and whisk together the 2 eggs.
- By adding the blended smooth mixture to the eggs whisks them together.
- Gradually add garlic and herb seasoning and salt until fully mixed in.
- When done, fold in the diced ham and spinach.
- Spray some cooking oil in a casserole and put the mixture in it.
- Bake it for 30-35 minutes at 350°F.

3. Classic Omelet

An age-old recipe to suit your taste bud any time.

Ingredients (4 servings)

- 12 eggs
- 4 tbsp. sour cream or heavy whipping cream
- 7 oz. shredded cheese
- 1 yellow onion, finely chopped
- 4¼ oz. butter
- ⅔ lb. ham, diced
- 1 finely chopped green bell pepper
- salt and pepper

Instructions

- Take a bowl and whisk cream and eggs together. Add salt and pepper to it.
- Add half of the cheese to the whisked mixture
- Melt butter in a frying pan and Sauté onion, ham and pepper diced in medium flame.
- When done add egg batter and fry till the omelet is done.
- After reducing the heat sprinkle the rest cheese over the omelet and it is ready to be served.

4. Avocado Eggs with Bacon Sails

If you have some extra time to make your breakfast try this and sail with your family!

Ingredients (2 servings)

- 2 hard-boiled eggs
- ½ avocado
- 2 oz. bacon
- 1 tsp. olive oil
- salt and pepper

Instructions

- Take eggs and half boil them. Cut the eggs from the middle.
- By scooping the yolk out from egg mash it with avocado, salt, pepper, and oil.
- Bake the bacon in a frying pan or in the oven for 5 to 7 minutes at 350°F.
- Take a spoon and put the mixture in the egg shell and with the fried or baked bacon prepare the sail.

5. Smoked Salmon Sandwich

A sandwich is the best food for breakfast and if it is with salmon nothing like it!

Ingredients (2 servings)

- 8 eggs
- 6⅓ oz. smoked salmon
- 4 tbsp. heavy whipping cream
- 2 oz. lettuce
- 2 pinches chili flakes
- 4 slices of low-carb bread
- 4¼ oz. butter for frying
- 4 tbsp. butter
- salt and pepper
- optional 2 tbsp. fresh chopped chives

Instructions

- Take a bowl and whisk eggs and cream in it. Add salt and pepper as required.
- Take frying pan and melt butter in it over medium heat. Add the egg mixture and stir it till it gets blended. When done remove from heat.
- Add chili to the mix. You can use chili flakes or finely chopped chilies too.
- Apply a thick layer of butter to the low carb bread and toast it.
- In between the bread slices put a few lettuce leaves, scrambled eggs, and smoked salmon. If you wish you can add chives that are chopped finely.

6. Green eggs

A great way to start your day in a green way.

Ingredients (4 servings)

- 8 eggs
- 8 leaves of kale along with stems
- Pinch of Celtic sea salt
- Oil for frying

Instructions

- Put kale, eggs, and salt in a blender and blend till it is smooth.
- Add oil in a frying pan and heat it in medium flame.
- Pour the blended mixture into the frying pan.
- Cook the egg to your preferred doneness.

7. Keto Bread Loaves

While on a Ketogenic diet you will need bread either to eat them separately or with some other recipe.

Ingredients (8 servings)

- 6 eggs
- 1 cup sifted coconut flour
- ½ cup water
- ½ cup flaxseed meal
- 1 Tbsp. apple cider vinegar
- 1 tsp. baking powder
- 1 tsp. salt
- ½ tsp. baking soda

Instructions

- Take a mixing bowl and sift coconut flour in it.
- In the meantime, preheat the oven at 350ºF and grease the pan.
- Add other ingredients in the mixing bowl and whisk them together.
- Add till the better is thick and comes together.
- Put the batter in the greased pan and bake it for about 40 minutes.
- Let the bread cool and then remove it from pan.

8. Low Carb Irish Colcannon

Enjoy this Irish dish made with kale and cauliflower to start your day in a healthy way.

Ingredients (6 servings)

- 1 cup frozen thawed spinach
- 3 cups cauliflower florets
- 1/2 medium avocado
- 1/4 cup cream
- 4 Tbsp. butter
- 1/2 cup sour cream
- 1/2 tsp. salt
- Fresh black pepper

Instructions

- Put cauliflower and spinach in a bowl and cook them till the cauliflower becomes tender.
- Add avocado, cream, butter, seasonings and sour cream to the boiled mix and put them in a blender.
- Blend them until its smooth. You can add some black pepper and salt as per your taste.
- Top colcannon with some sour cream.

9. Sage and Cheddar Waffles

Waffles are always a great way to start your day. You can enjoy them as breakfast or treat.

Ingredients (4 servings)

- 1 $^{1/3}$ cup sifted coconut flour
- 2 cups canned coconut milk
- 1 tsp. dried ground sage
- 3 tsp. baking powder
- ¼ tsp. garlic powder
- ½ tsp. salt
- 2 eggs
- 3 Tbsp. coconut oil, melted
- ½ cup water
- 1 cup cheddar cheese, shredded

Instructions

- Heat your waffle iron at moderate temperature.
- Take a mixing bowl and whisk flour, seasonings and baking powder.
- Now add the liquid ingredients like coconut milk. Stir it till the batter is stiff.
- Add cheese to the mixture.
- Grease the waffles iron on both sides and pour part of batter into it.
- Close the iron and wait till steam rises.

10. Keto Breakfast Brownie Muffins

Want something that can keep you filled till lunch time. Enjoy these muffins.

Ingredients (3 servings)

- 1 cup Golden Flaxseed Meal
- 1/4 cup Cocoa Powder
- 1/4 cup Sugar-free Caramel Syrup
- 1 tbsp. Cinnamon
- 1/2 tbsp. Baking Powder
- 1 large Egg
- 1/2 tsp. Salt
- 1 tsp. Vanilla Extract
- 2 tbsp. Coconut Oil
- 1/2 cup Pumpkin Puree
- 1/4 cup Slivered Almonds
- 1 tsp. Apple Cider Vinegar

Instructions

- Preheat your oven to 350°F.
- Take a deep mixing bowl and combine all ingredients in it.
- Take a muffin tin and line it with 6 paper liners.
- Put around ¼ cup of batter into the muffin tins.
- Sprinkle some almonds over the mixture.
- Bake it for 15 minutes and then remove and serve.

11. Keto Breakfast Tacos

On your ketogenic diets, tacos can be good for hands on attitude.

Ingredients (3 servings)

- 6 large Eggs
- 1 cup shredded Mozzarella Cheese
- 3 strips Bacon
- 2 tbsp. Butter
- 1 oz. shredded Cheddar Cheese
- 1/2 small Avocado
- Salt and Pepper to Taste

Instructions

- First, cook the bacon for about 15 to 20 minutes at 375°F.
- While the bacon is cooking heat about 1/3 cup of mozzarella on a clean pan.
- Wait for about 2 to 3 minutes till the cheese is browned.
- Using a pair of tongs lift the shell up. Then drape it on a wooden spatula. Carry this on for the rest of cheese. This way you can make the tacos shell.
- Take eggs and cook it in butter. Keep stirring till they are done. Season them with pepper and salt.
- In the hardened taco shell pours in the avocado, scrambled egg, and bacon.
- Sprinkle some cheddar cheese over the tacos and they are ready to serve.

12. Keto Breakfast Burger

This is a fantastic option for a heavy breakfast or a brunch

Ingredients (2 servings)

- 2 large Eggs
- 4 oz. Sausage
- 2 oz. Pepper jack Cheese
- 4 slices Bacon
- 1 tbsp. PB Fit Powder
- 1 tbsp. Butter
- Salt and Pepper

Instructions

- Take bacon and cook it in the oven for 20 to 25 minutes at 400F
- Mix PB Fit powder and butter in a bowl and set aside.
- Make sausage patties and cook them on both sides. Add cheese to the patties and cover them with lids.
- Remove from pan and serve.

13. Tuna Salad with Capers

Start your day with Tuna salad along with capers, a perfect Keto breakfast.

Ingredients (4 servings)

- 1 can tuna in olive oil
- 2 tbsp. sour cream
- 8 tbsp. mayonnaise
- 3 – 5 finely chopped leeks
- chili flakes, to taste
- 1 Tbsp. capers
- salt and pepper

Instructions

- Drain the Tuna.
- Mix all the ingredients together and season it with salt and pepper.
- If required you can sprinkle chili flakes. Serve with boiled eggs.

14. Dairy-Free Latte

When in hurry in the morning have this to complete your breakfast.

Ingredients (2 servings)

- 4 large eggs
- 4 tbsp. coconut oil
- 2 pinches vanilla extract
- 3⅓ cups boiling water
- 2 tsp. s ground ginger or pumpkin pie spice

Instructions

- Blend all ingredients with a stick blender.
- Drink immediately.

15. Bulletproof Coffee

A Warm, filling and delicious start to your day!

Ingredients (2 servings)

- 2 tbsp. coconut oil
- 2 cups hot coffee freshly brewed
- 2 tbsp. unsalted butter

Instructions

- Mix all ingredients in a blender until frothy and smooth.
- Serve immediately.

Chapter 4.2

Keto Lunch Recipes

Whether you are busy during the afternoon or just want to enjoy a good meal here is a collection of few best keto lunch recipes.

16. Keto Okonomiyaki

Okonomiyaki is a pancake that is stuffed with shredded cabbage and meat.

Ingredients (3 servings)

For Batter

- 1 large egg
- 1 Tbsp. butter softened
- 1 Tbsp. softened cream cheese
- ½ tsp. baking powder
- 1 Tbsp. flax meal
- 2 tbsp. almond flour
- ¼ tsp. salt

Filling

- 3 ounces' green cabbage, shredded
- 2 slices thickly sliced bacon

Toppings

- ¼ cup mayonnaise
- 1 Tbsp. bonito flakes

- 1 ½ tbsp. sugar-free BBQ Sauce
- 1 tsp. unseasoned rice vinegar
- ½ Tbsp. seaweed flakes

Instructions

- Preheat a skillet. Make a sauce by mixing ¼ cup of mayo and unseasoned rice vinegar. If possible load the sauce in a bottle.
- In a mixing bowl add butter and cream cheese. Then add flax meal, almond flour, baking powder, and salt to the batter.
- Form a smooth batter by stirring the mixture gently.
- Add egg in the mixture and keep stirring till it is fully incorporated.
- Put the cabbage in the batter and coat each cabbage properly.
- Cut the bacon into square slices and fry them in the skillet.
- After the bacon is crispy on one side flip it over. You should arrange them in the center of the skillet. Normally the bacon will kick off oil so you may not require doing so. If needed you can add some.
- Take the okonomiyaki batter and spread it over the bacon to form a pancake.
- Cover the skillet with a lid and let it cook for about 5 to 7 minutes.

- If the bacon and the butter are brown on one side you can flip it over. If required add some oil.
- Transfer the pancake to a plate and spread BBQ sauce over it.
- Squeeze mayo and make it design.
- Finally, top it with bonito flakes and serve after cutting the pancake.

17. Savory Italian Egg Bake

This easy Italian bake is a combination of delicious tastes of broccoli, chicken, and cheese

Ingredients (8 servings)

- 10 large eggs
- 2 tsp. herb and garlic seasoning
- 3 tbsp. mustard
- ½ cup tomato sauce
- ½ cup heavy whipping cream
- 1 tsp. parsley flakes
- 12 ounces' frozen broccoli florets
- 2 cups diced chicken breast, cooked
- ½ cup Parmesan cheese, grated
- 1 cup extra sharp cheese, shredded

Instructions

- Preheat oven to 350°F.
- Whisk the eggs together in a mixing bowl.
- Add garlic, mustard, herbs and heavy whipping cream.
- After all, this is blended nicely add the tomato sauce and whisk it slowly so that no lumps are formed.
- Add in the broccoli florets and diced chicken.
- The Italian bake is ready so pour it in a large baking dish.

- Sprinkle some parsley flakes and parmesan cheese over the bake. Bake it for 30 to 40 minutes at 350°F.
- Before serving you can add some more cheese as topping to make it perfect Keto.

18. Sausage and Kale Soup

Enjoy this Keto soup and get the essence of Italian savory right at your bowl.

Ingredients (6 servings)

- 1 lb. ground sweet Italian sausage
- 1 medium chopped yellow onion
- 1 Tbsp. butter
- 2 tbsp. red wine vinegar
- 1 tsp. dried rubbed sage
- 1 medium peeled and diced carrot
- 2 cloves garlic, crushed
- 4 cups low-sodium chicken broth
- 1 tsp. dried basil
- 1 tsp. dried oregano
- 1 cup heavy cream
- ½ medium head cauliflower
- 3 cups chopped kale
- ¼ tsp. crushed red pepper flakes
- Sea salt
- ½ tsp. black pepper

Instructions

- Heat a large saucepan and add sausage to it. Cook it by stirring occasionally until it turns brown.
- Remove the cooked sausages and drain them on a plate.

- In the same pan melt butter. After the bubbling reduces add carrots and onions to it. Cook them till the onion becomes translucent.
- Add garlic to the pan and cook for one minute. Add red wine vinegar. It will become syrupy that will scrape brown bits.
- Stir in oregano, sage, basil and red pepper flakes and add heavy cream and stock to it.
- After the soup reaches simmer add cauliflower and let it simmer more.
- Then add the cooked sausages and kale.
- Wait till all the ingredients become tender. Season it with salt and pepper.

19. Apple and Ham Flatbread

Try this flatbread recipe and enjoy!

Ingredients (2 servings)

For the crust

- 2 cups grated part-skim mozzarella cheese
- 2 Tbsp. cream cheese
- ¾ cup almond flour
- 1/8 tsp. dried thyme
- ½ tsp. sea salt

For the topping

- 1 cup grated Mexican cheese
- ½ small red onion
- ¼ medium apple
- 1/8 tsp. dried thyme
- 4 oz. sliced ham
- Salt and Pepper

Instructions

- Slice the red onions thinly, remove the core from apple and slice them thinly after peeling it. Cut the sliced ham into square chunks.
- Preheat oven to 425º Fahrenheit. Also, have a pizza pan and a rolling pin ready. Cut two parchment papers into 2 inches bigger than the pizza pan.

- Fill a sauce pot partially with water and put a mixing bowl fitting the top. It will act as a double boiler. Bring water in the pot to simmer over high heat and then turn it to low.
- In the double boiler, mixing bowl add cream cheese, mozzarella cheese, thyme, almond flour, and salt. By putting the bowl over the simmering pot keeps stirring constantly.
- As the cheese will melt the ingredients will hold together and you can make the dough. Dump it over a parchment paper.
- Knead the dough so that it mixes thoroughly.
- Now after rolling the dough into a ball put it on the parchment paper. Take a rolling pin and roll the dough into a circle.
- Put it on the pizza pan along with the parchment paper. Use a fork to poke holes in the dough. Bake it in the oven for 6-8 minutes. When it's golden brown remove it.
- Sprinkle some cheese over the flatbread, and then arrange the apple slices and the onion slices. Layer the ham pieces on it.
- Cover it with the rest cheese. Spread thyme, black pepper, and salt over the cheese.
- Bake it at 350°F till the crust becomes golden brown or for about 5 to 7 minutes.

20. Avocado Tuna Melt Bites

These keto melt bites are crispy outside and creamy inside that makes your meal outstanding.

Ingredients (12 pieces)

- 10 oz. drained canned Tuna
- 1 medium cubed Avocado
- 1/4 cup Mayonnaise
- 1/3 cup Almond Flour
- 1/4 cup Parmesan Cheese
- 1/4 tsp. Onion Powder
- 1/2 tsp. Garlic Powder
- Salt and Pepper
- 1/2 cup Coconut Oil, for frying

Instructions

- Take a mixing bowl and add tuna along with all ingredients. Leave the avocado and coconut oil.
- Fold the tuna around the avocado tubes.
- Form tuna balls and cover it with almond flour.
- Heat coconut oil in a pan and fry the tuna balls till they are brown. Serve hot with dip.

21. Keto Mixed Green Spring Salad

The salad is always a great helping for anytime. During lunch, it is indeed filling.

Ingredients (1 serving)

- 2 oz. Mixed Greens
- 2 tbsp. Shaved Parmesan
- 3 tbsp. roasted Pine Nuts
- 2 slices Bacon
- 2 tbsp. Raspberry Vinaigrette
- Salt and Pepper

Instructions

- Take a pan and cook bacon on it till its crispy.
- Crumble the bacon and add it to the salad along with other ingredients.
- Mix the salad and serve.

22. 5 Minute Keto Egg Drop Soup

When in hurry prepare this egg drop soup and enjoy your lunch.

Ingredients (2 servings)

- 2 large Eggs
- 1 1/2 cups Chicken Broth
- 1 tbsp. Bacon Fat
- 1/2 cube Chicken Bouillon
- 1 tsp. Chili Garlic Paste

Instructions

- Heat a pan on the stove and heat it in medium flame. Put in the bullion cubes, bacon fat, chicken broth.
- Add the mixture and then bring the broth to boil.
- Add and stir the chili garlic paste and turn off the stove.
- In the steaming broth pour beaten eggs and keep stirring during the process.
- Let it sit for some time and serve.

23. Ketogenic Nasi Lemak

This popular rice dish of Malaysia, Singapore, Indonesia and Brunei is a perfect ketogenic lunch recipe.

Ingredients (2 servings)

Fried Chicken

- 2 boneless Chicken Thighs
- 1/2 tsp. Lime Juice
- 1/4 tsp. Turmeric Powder
- 1/2 tsp. Curry Powder
- 1/2 tsp. Coconut Oil
- 1/8 tsp. Salt

Nasi Lemak

- 3 tbsp. Coconut Milk
- 3 slices Ginger
- 1/2 small sliced Shallot
- 4 slices Cucumber
- 7 oz. riced Cauliflower
- 1/4 tsp. Salt

Fried Egg

- 1 large Egg
- 1/2 tbsp. Butter Unsalted

Instructions

- Use a food processor to rice the cauliflower and then squeeze out the water.
- Take chicken thighs and marinate it with lime juice, turmeric powder, curry powder, and salt.
- Heat oil in a pan and fry the marinated chicken.
- Take a saucepan and boil coconut milk, shallots, and ginger. Once it starts bubbling add the cauliflower rice. Mix it well.
- In another frying pan pour unsalted butter and fry the eggs.
- Serve it with fried egg, fried chicken and 2 slices of cucumber.

24. Keto Pigs in a Blanket

It tastes as fancier as the name is. Serve it to your friends or enjoy it yourself.

Ingredients (37 pieces)

- 37 Little Smokies
- 2 cups Cheddar Cheese
- 1 tbsp. Psyllium Husk Powder
- 3/4 cup Almond Flour
- 1 large Egg
- 3 Tbsp. Cream Cheese
- 1/2 tsp. Salt and pepper.

Instructions

- Separate the wet and dry ingredients.
- Put the cheddar cheese in a microwave bowl and melt it till it starts bubbling.
- Mix all the ingredients except the smokies to form a dough.
- Preheat oven at 400°F
- Spread the dough in such manner on the Silpat that it fills up the total sheet. For hardening put it inside the freezer.
- After the dough is a cold transfer it to foil and cut it. Make out strips from the dough and wrap the strips around the smokies.
- Bake it in the oven for about 13 to 15 minutes.

25. Low-Carb Salmon Pie

Looking for an all in one dish for lunch? Try this recipe and you will be surprised and feel filled after you complete your meal.

Ingredients (4 servings)

Pie crust

- 1 egg
- ¾ cup almond flour
- 4 tbsp. coconut flour
- 4 tbsp. Sesame seeds
- 1 tsp. baking powder
- 1 Tbsp. ground psyllium husk powder
- 3 tbsp. olive oil or coconut oil
- 1 pinch salt
- 4 tbsp. water

Filling

- 3 eggs
- ½ lb. smoked salmon
- 2 tbsp. finely chopped fresh dill
- 1 cup mayonnaise
- ¼ tsp. ground black pepper
- ½ tsp. onion powder
- 1¼ cups shredded cheese
- 4¼ oz. cream cheese

Instructions

- Take all the ingredients for the pie crust and pit them in your food processor. As the dough is form remove it.
- Preheat the oven to 350°F
- For removing the pie when it is done attach a piece of parchment paper along with a spring form. It becomes easier to remove the crust.
- Take the dough from the food processor and spread it on the form. For spreading you can use your fingers or use a spatula.
- Pre-bake the crust for about 10-15 minutes.
- Take all ingredients of filling except the salmon and mix it well.
- Pour the mixture into the pie crust.
- Add salmon over the mixture and bake it for about 35 minutes.
- Take out once the pie has great color and serve.

Chapter 4.3

Keto Dinner Recipes

It is said that dinner is the most important meal of the day. Even when following a ketogenic diet plan, you should have filling dinner so that you can start your next day energized. Looking for something tasty yet healthy dinner recipes? Here are they

26. Salad in a Jar

A healthy way to enjoy dinner and quick way to pack it. If you are going out during dinner carry it along with you and enjoy the delicious salad along with chicken or salmon.

Ingredients (4 servings)

- 7¾ oz. rotisserie or chickens smoked salmon or any other protein of your choice
- 2 oz. cherry tomatoes
- 2 oz. leafy greens
- 2 oz. cucumber
- 2 oz. red bell peppers
- 8 tbsp. mayonnaise or olive oil
- 1 scallion

Instructions

- Take vegetables of your choice and start putting them in the jar in layers.
- Take the dark leafy vegetables like arugula or spinach and put them in the bottom of the jar.
- You can add layers of different vegetables like the red cabbages make a good impression, chopped cauliflower or broccoli is healthy and lettuce are good too.
- Keep on adding other ingredients like shredded carrot, sliced onion rings, avocado, bell peppers and tomato in different layers.
- For topping the salad, grilled chicken or smoked salmon is mentioned. You can choose any other form of protein like boiled eggs, canned tuna or something else.
- You may add nuts, olives or cheese cubes to add in the fat.
- Right before serving pour in some mayonnaise in the salad and its perfect.

27. Keto Sweet and Sour Meatballs

Just like Chinese sweet and sour chicken these meatballs are always a loved item when served in dinner.

Ingredients (5 servings)

The meatballs

- 1 large egg
- 1 pound ground beef
- ½ tsp. onion powder
- ¼ cup Parmesan cheese

For the sauce

- ¼ cup apple cider vinegar
- 1 ½ cups water
- 1 cup sugar-free ketchup
- 3 tbsp. soy sauce
- ½ tsp. xanthan gum
- 1 cup erythritol

Instructions

- Add ground beef, grated parmesan cheese, an egg and onion powder in a mixing bowl. Mix the ingredients properly with hands.
- The mixture for meatballs is ready. Take a tablespoon and shape the meatballs. You should be able to shape at least 30 meatballs.
- Preheat a saucepan and put oil in it. Put the meatballs and cook until they are brown outside. If they are a little bit pink in the middle no issues, keep them aside.
- Tae the same saucepan and add apple cider vinegar, water, sugar-free ketchup, soy sauce and erythritol. Stir the mixture completely till the sauce comes together.
- Slowly whisk the xanthan gum in the mixture. Let it thicken and in the meantime, keep stirring the mixture. Simmer the sauce in low temperature.
- Simmer the sauce till you get the desired consistency. You can try out a spoon to understand if you have got the desired consistency.
- If you find the sauce perfect them add the meatballs into it and let it simmer for few more minutes.
- Serve hot when the meatballs are cooked properly.

28. Garlic Chicken

A common and simple recipe changed a bit to serve it as Ketogenic meal. The garlic along with chicken makes the perfect combination.

Ingredients (4 servings)

- 2¼ lbs. chicken thighs
- 5 to 10 sliced garlic cloves
- 2 tbsp. olive oil
- 4 tbsp. butter
- 8 tbsp. finely chopped fresh parsley
- 1 lemon, the juice

Instructions

- Preheat the oven to about 450°F.
- Take a baking pan and grease it with butter. Place the chicken pieces on it.
- Pour in salt and pepper as per taste over the chicken pieces.
- Also, sprinkle parsley and garlic and drizzle some lemon juice. Pour olive oil on the top.
- Bake the chicken until its golden brown. The garlic slices must have been roasted and turned brown.
- It may take about 30 to 50 minutes depending upon the size of the chicken pieces.

29. Creamy Keto Shrimp Tacos

It's not that the taco fillings are only interesting. This keto recipe it's the cheesy taco shells that attract most and the shrimps add to the delicious taste.

Ingredients (4 servings)

Taco shells

- ½ tsp. ground cumin
- ½ lb. shredded cheese

Creamy shrimp filling

- 2/3 lb. peeled shrimps
- 2 tbsp. coconut oil
- 2 finely chopped garlic cloves
- ½ lime, the juice
- 1 finely chopped red chili pepper that is deseeded
- 1 cup mayonnaise
- 4 tbsp. chopped fresh cilantro
- 1 tomato, finely chopped
- 1 avocado, diced
- salt, and pepper

Instructions

- For preparing the taco shells to mix the cumin and the cheese.
- Preheat the oven to 400°F.
- With the mixture of cumin and cheese from about eight piles on the baking sheet that is lined with parchment paper.
- There should be enough space between the piles so that the cheese does not melt and mix with each other.
- Put the baking tray in the oven and bake in for 10 to 15 minutes till the cheese is bubbling. Make sure that the cheese is not burned as it will not taste good.
- Place the racks over a sink and place the cheese rounds on the racks carefully.
- Once it is cooled you can fill the tacos with any filling of your choice.
- For making the creamy shrimp filling, sauté the shrimp on hot pan and pour some coconut oil in the pan.
- Add garlic and chilli and sauté the mixture till the shrimp changes its color to pink.
- Add salt to taste.
- Take all other ingredients in a mixing bowl and add them together with the fried shrimps.
- Mix them well and fill the tacos with the creamy filling. Serve immediately.

30. Mushroom Omelet

The mushroom omelet is preferred by many as breakfast, but taking it during dinner is also good. Try it out and enjoy the taste of mushrooms.

Ingredients (4 servings)

- 6 eggs
- 1¾ oz. shredded cheese
- 1¾ oz. butter, for frying
- 4 - 6 mushrooms
- 2⁄5 yellow onion
- salt and pepper

Instructions

- Take a mixing bowl and crack the eggs in it. Add a pinch of salt and pepper as per your taste and whisk it with a fork. Whisk till it becomes frothy and smooth.
- Add rest of spices and salt
- Take a frying pan and melt the butter in it.
- Once the butter is melted pour in the egg mixture inside it.
- As the omelet begins to cook but is still raw add mushroom, cheese and onions one by one.
- Take a spatula and carefully fold the edges of the omelet and fold it half.
- Once the color changes to golden brown slide the omelet to a plate and serves hot.

31. Meatballs

Meatballs are the perfect company to any meal. They are high in fat and low carb. They also contain required protein so a perfect ketogenic dish.

Ingredients (12 pieces)

- 1 pound ground beef
- 1 minced shallot
- 1 large egg
- 2 tbsp. Dijon mustard
- 2 tbsp. tomato paste
- ½ tsp. ground black pepper
- 1 Tbsp. coconut flour
- ¼ tsp. baking soda
- ½ tsp. Celtic sea salt

Instructions

- In a large bowl take eggs, ground beef, and shallot and combine them well.
- Add in tomato paste, coconut flour, mustard, baking soda, salt, and pepper.
- Mix all the ingredients firmly.
- Form meatballs with the mixture. You can make the ¼-cup scoop.
- Take a parchment lined baking sheet and place the meatballs over it.
- Bake the meatballs at 350°F for about 30 minutes
- Serve along with zucchini noodles or spaghetti noodles along with the marinara sauce.

32. Beef Brisket

A recipe to make your dinner a celebration.

Ingredients (1 serving)

- 1½ pounds brisket, stew meat or shoulder roast, flank rib
- 1 chopped large onion
- 3 cups chicken stock
- 8 sliced carrots
- 8 cloves peeled and sliced garlic
- 8 ounces sliced mushrooms,
- 1 Tbsp. onion powder
- 1 Tbsp. garlic powder
- ½ tsp. Celtic sea salt

Instructions

- Take a crockpot and place stock, garlic, onion, carrots and mushrooms.
- Sprinkle some onion powder, garlic powder and salt in the crockpot.
- Place the meat in the center.
- Turn on the crockpot and low heat and let it cook till 6 to 8 hours.
- Serve it hot when done.

33. Salmon Wasabi Burgers

If you want something extra during your dinner try this out. You will enjoy the taste and its filling too!

Ingredients (4 Servings)

- 1 pound skinless salmon filet
- ¼ cup finely chopped fresh scallions
- 2 large eggs
- 1 Tbsp. fresh ginger
- ¼ cup minced fresh cilantro
- ½ cup blanched almond flour
- ¼ cup wasabi powder
- coconut oil for frying
- 1 Tbsp. freshly squeezed lime juice
- 1 tsp. Celtic sea salt
- 1 Tbsp. water

Instructions

- Take the ginger and peel them off and mince them.
- Rinse the salmon and pat them dry. Then cut them into cubes.
- Take a large bowl and combine salmon, scallions, ginger, cilantro, eggs, almond flour, lime juice, and salt.
- In another small bowl form a paste by combining wasabi and water.
- Mix the wasabi paste along with the salmon mixture.
- With your hands form a batter of 2 inches' patties.
- Heat oil for frying and put the patties. Fry them till golden brown and serve hot.

34. Perfect Roast Chicken

Roast chicken is perfect dinner recipe that can be enjoyed along with your family or when guests are there.

Ingredients (for single chicken)

- 1 whole chicken of 2-3 pounds
- freshly ground black pepper
- Celtic sea salt
- 1 in head garlic, cut half crosswise
- 1 lemon, halved
- 1 bunch fresh thyme
- 1 medium onion, quartered
- 2 tbsp. olive oil

Instructions

- Preheat oven to 425°
- Clean the chicken and rinse it outside and in thoroughly.
- Take a 9x13 baking dish and place the chicken over it.
- Sprinkle salt and pepper over the chicken.
- Stuff in the cavity with both halves of lemon, a bunch of thyme and garlic.
- Brush olive oil on the chicken and sprinkle some salt and pepper.
- Tuck the wings under the body of the chicken and tie the legs together with kitchen string.
- In the corner of the dish place onions
- Roast the chicken for about 1 and ½ hour and serve after cooling slightly.

35. Grilled Salmon Paprika

Ingredients (single serving)

- 1½ pound salmon fillet
- 1 Tbsp. smoked paprika
- ¼ cup honey or agave nectar
- ½ tsp. ground cumin
- 1 tsp. Celtic sea salt

Instructions

- The salmon should be cut into 4 ounces' pieces. Rinse the fish, pat it dry and place it on the 7x11 inch baking dish.
- Take a small bowl and combine cumin, paprika, and salt in it
- Drizzle some agave or honey over the salmon and then sprinkle the paprika mixture.
- Marinate it for about 5 hours at least
- Grill the salmon for about 4 to 5 minutes and turn.
- Grill the other side and its ready to be served.

36. Stuffed Peppers

You can stuff the peppers with anything, we have used turkey here.

Ingredients (3 servings)

- 6-8 sweet bell peppers (orange, green, yellow or red)
- 1 pound ground turkey
- 4 oz. diced green chilies
- 1 cup finely chopped cilantro
- 2 tsp. cumin
- ½ cup finely chopped onion
- 1 tsp. chili powder
- 1 tsp. Celtic sea salt

Instructions

- Take a medium size bowl and mix diced chiles with turkey, onion, cilantro, cumin, salt and chili powder.
- Take different colored bell peppers and cut off the top. Keep them aside.
- Place the peppers in 7x11 inch baking dish.
- Stuff the turkey mixture in the peppers. Close the peppers with tops.
- Bake at 350° for 1 hour and Serve

37. Cobb Salad

Ingredients

- 1 pound cooked chicken breast, small size
- 1 cup sliced cherry tomatoes
- 6 large romaine lettuce leaves
- 1 diced avocado
- 8 cooked pieces bacon
- 4 sliced into quarters large hard boiled eggs
- Homemade Ranch Dressing, to taste

Instructions

- Take the chicken breast and dice them into ½-inch cubes.
- Cut thin slices of lettuce and place them on plates.
- Top the lettuce with chicken, avocados, and tomatoes.
- Crumble the crisp bacon and sprinkle it over the salad.
- Drizzle some ranch dressings and serve.

38. Turkey Bean Chili

Ingredients (4 servings)

- 2 tbsp. olive oil
- 1 diced onion
- 1 thinly sliced clove garlic
- 1 sliced pint cherry tomatoes
- 1 Tbsp. dried oregano
- 1 cup water
- ½ tsp. Celtic sea salt
- ½ tsp. chili powder
- 1 lb. ground turkey
- 1 cup beans

Instructions

- Soak the beans overnight and cook them.
- Heat olive oil in a large skillet.
- Add onion to the oil and sauté for 10minutes.
- Add cherry tomatoes, garlic, water, chili, oregano, and salt.
- Cover the skillet and cook till the tomatoes are soft enough to fall apart.
- Add turkey meat to the skillet and cook for another 10 minutes.
- Add in the beans along with the cooking juice.
- It is ready to serve.

39. Mango Chicken

A different flavor of chicken to be served right at the dinner table.

Ingredients (5 servings)

- 1 ¼ pounds chicken breast
- ¼ cup olive oil or grapeseed oil
- 1 diced red bell pepper
- 1 large onion
- 1 tsp. curry powder
- 2 sliced garlic cloves
- 1 Tbsp. apple cider vinegar
- 1 Tbsp. minced fresh ginger
- ½ cup full fat coconut milk
- 1 tsp. Celtic sea salt
- 1 cup water
- 1 peeled and diced mango

Instructions

- Cut the chicken breast into 1-inch cubes.
- Warm oil in a large sauté pan. Add onion to the pan and stir occasionally till the onion softens.
- Add red pepper, garlic, ginger, curry and salt, and cook for 5 minutes
- Add vinegar, coconut milk, water, and mango to the pan. Bring the mixture to boil and then reduce the heat.
- Add chicken pieces, and reduce the heat so that the mixture simmers.
- Cook for about 10 to 15 minutes till the chicken is cooked. Serve hot.

40. Fish Sticks

Ingredients (4 servings)

- 1 pound white fish (such as snapper, cod, or tilapia)
- 1 cup blanched almond flour
- 2 large whisked eggs
- 6 tbsp. coconut oil or olive oil
- 1 tsp. Celtic sea salt

Instructions

- Rinse the fish fillet nicely and place them on a plate.
- Place the eggs in one bowl and flour and salt mixture in another.
- Dip the fish sticks in eggs and then in the flour. Place them on a plate.
- Heat oil in a skillet and place the fish sticks in the oil. They should not be crowded or else they will stick with each other.
- Cook for few minutes till the fish sticks turn brown on both sides.
- Transfer on a paper towel before serving it with sauce.

Chapter 4.4

Keto Snacks recipes

You will need food at a regular interval in your ketogenic diet plan, hence, you also must have a reserve of some delicious Keto snacks that are easy to prepare and tasty to eat.

41. Cheese Chips

Want something to enjoy with your favorite dip, try these chips.

Ingredients (4 servings)

- ½ lb. cheddar cheese or Edam cheese or provolone cheese
- ½ tsp. paprika powder

Instructions

- Preheat the oven to 400°F.
- Take the cheese slices and place them on a baking sheet lined with parchment paper.
- Sprinkle some paprika powder and start baking. Bake it for about 8 to 10 minutes.
- Make sure that the cheese slices do not burn as they will turn bitter.
- Cool it and enjoy with your favorite dip.

42. Raspberry Lemon Popsicles

Ingredient (6 servings)

- 100g Raspberries
- 1/4 cup Coconut Oil
- Juice 1/2 Lemon
- 1/4 cup Sour Cream
- 1 cup Coconut Milk
- 1/2 tsp. Guar Gum
- 1/4 cup Heavy Cream
- 20 drops Liquid Stevia

Instructions

- Take a container and add all the ingredients. By using an immersion blender blend the ingredients till they are smooth.
- Strain the mixture so that you can discard the raspberry seeds.
- Take molds and pour the mixture in it. Freeze them for at least 2 hours.
- Once the mixture has hardened run the mold under water to dislodge the popsicles. You may use hot water.

43. Jalapeno Popper Fat Bombs

These fat bombs contain enough fat to energize you the whole day.

Ingredients (4 servings)

- 3 slices Bacon
- 3 oz. Cream Cheese
- 1/2 tsp. Dried Parsley
- 1 medium Jalapeno Pepper
- 1/4 tsp. Garlic Powder
- 1/4 tsp. Onion Powder
- Salt and Pepper

Instructions

- Fry the bacon slices in a skillet till they are crispy. Set aside and put them on paper towels.
- Take jalapeno pepper and de-seed it. Dice the peppers into small pieces.
- Mix them together with bacon fat, cream cheese, and spices.
- Crumble the bacon and set them on a plate. Roll the cream cheese mixture into balls.
- Then roll these balls into bacon and they are ready to serve.

44. Keto Chocolate Chunk Cookies

Not only children but you too will love chocolate. Try these chocolate cookies and get indulge in your childhood.

Ingredients (16 pieces)

- 1 cup Almond Flour
- 2 tbsp. Coconut Flour
- 3 tbsp. Unflavored Whey Protein
- 8 tbsp. Unsalted Butter
- 2 tbsp. Psyllium Husk
- 1/4 cup Erythritol
- 2 tsp. Vanilla Extract
- 1/2 tsp. Baking Powder
- 10 drops Liquid Stevia
- 5 bars Cocoa Bar
- 1 large Egg

Instructions

- Take the dry ingredients and mix them together.
- Preheat oven at 350°F.
- Beat the butter until it is light in color, and then add stevia and erythritol. Beat it again.
- Add egg and vanilla extract and again beat the mixture.
- Gradually sift the dry ingredients over the wet ingredients and mix them together.
- Chop the cocoa bars into chunks and mix it into the dough. Roll the dough and cut out 16 pieces.
- Roll dough into balls and by placing them on Silpat press it with the base of Mason jar.
- Bake them for about 12 to 15 minutes.
- Serve when cool.

45. Salami and Cheese Chips

Loved Cheese chips, try this out too, a great combination.

Ingredients (4 servings)

- 4½ oz. grated parmesan cheese
- 3¼ oz. salami, about 20 slices
- 1 tsp. paprika powder

Instructions

- Preheat the oven to 450°F. Also put the broil function on.
- Take a baking sheet lined with parchment paper and place the salami slices over it. Always allow some space between the slices.
- On the top of every slice place a mound of shredded cheese.
- Sprinkle paprika powder and if you want the additional flavor you can sprinkle dry herbs too.
- Place the dish in the oven and bake till the cheese turns bubbly.
- Let them cool after removing from the oven. It's time to enjoy it!

46. Goat Cheese Tomato Tarts

With some extra effort, you can astonish your guests who think that as you are in the ketogenic diet you are on a restrictive diet!

Ingredients (12 pieces)

Roasted Tomatoes

- 2 medium Tomatoes
- 1/4 cup Olive Oil
- Salt & Pepper

Tart Base

- 2 tbsp. Coconut Flour
- 1 tbsp. Psyllium Husk
- 1/2 cup Almond Flour
- 5 tbsp. Cold Butter, Cubed
- 1/4 tsp. Salt

Tart Filling

- 1/2 medium thinly sliced Onion,
- 3 oz. Goat Cheese
- 2 tsp. Minced Garlic
- 2 tbsp. Olive Oil
- 3 tsp. fresh Thyme

Instructions

- Pre-heat the oven at 435 °F. Take the tomatoes and slice them into 1/4", then drizzle some olive oil over it. You can season it with salt and pepper.
- Put the tomatoes in the oven and roast them for 30 minutes. To minimize the steaming effect, you can poke small holes.
- For making the tart base, combine all tart base ingredients in the food processor. Pulse it slowly so that dough is made.
- By using silicone cupcake molds press the dough into thin layers. You will get around 12 tarts.
- Preheat the oven and bake the dough for 17 to 20 minutes. The tarts will harden and then its times to remove them from the oven. Let it cool down totally.
- You can remove the tart from the mold by tapping on the bottom of the cupcake mold.
- In a pan, caramelize the garlic and the onion in 2 tablespoon olive oil.
- Assemble the tarts with caramelized fillings, tomato, fresh thyme and crumbled goat cheese.
- Bake it at 350oF for around 6 to 7 minutes or till the cheese start melting.
- Remove it from oven and serve hot.

47. Cheese Roll-Ups

This is simple and fast low carb snacks. It is easy and tastes awesome.

Ingredients (4 servings)

- ½ lb. cheddar cheese or Edam cheese or provolone cheese
- optional seasoning of your choice
- 2 oz. butter

Instructions

- Place the cheese slices on a large cutting board. The cheese should be sliced.
- Slice butter with the cheese slice and cover each cheese slice with butter.
- Roll them and serve as snacks.

48. Cheese Puffs

Simple and fast cheese puffs are fast to make and tasty to eat.

Ingredients (3 servings)

- 1/3 lb. Brie cheese

Instructions

- Dice the brie cheese into ½ inch cubes. Do not forget to remove the white edges.
- Place the cheese cubes in parchment paper and bake it in the micro oven for about 1 to 2 minutes. Make sure that the cheese pieces do not get burnt.
- Let cool before serving.

49. Cinnamon and Cardamom Fat Bombs

They are small but delicious. Enjoy them as keto snacks.

Ingredients (4 servings)

- 1¾ oz. butter
- ½ pinch ground green cardamom
- 2 2/3 tbsp. unsweetened shredded coconut
- 1 pinch ground cinnamon
- 1/8 tsp. vanilla extract

Instructions

- The butter should be at room temperature.
- Take a pan and roast the shredded coconut until it turns brownish.
- Take a bowl and mix together the butter, spices, and half of the shredded coconut.
- Take the mixture in hand and form a walnut size balls.
- Roll the balls in the rest shredded coconut.
- Put them in the freezer and serve cool.

50. Hot Deviled Eggs

Looking for a low carb recipe for Halloween? Here it is, enjoy your Halloween or other holidays.

Ingredients (4 servings)

- 4 eggs
- 1/3 cup mayonnaise
- 2/3 Tbsp. red curry paste
- 1/3 Tbsp. poppy seeds
- 1/6 tsp. salt

Instructions

- Boil the eggs in water for about 8 minutes. After that put them in ice cold water.
- Remove the egg shells and split the egg into equal halves.
- Scoop out the egg yolk and place it in a small bowl.
- Place the egg whites on a plate and set aside in the refrigerator.
- Form a smooth batter with mayonnaise, curry paste, and egg yolks.
- Put the batter in the egg whites.
- Sprinkle some poppy seeds on the top and serve!

51. Cheddar Cheese and Bacon Balls

Cheese and bacon! A lovely combination. This awe-inspiring keto snack is easy and simple to make

Ingredients (4 servings)

- 2⅔ oz. bacon
- 2⅔ oz. cream cheese
- ½ Tbsp. butter
- 1 oz. butter
- 2⅔ oz. cheddar cheese
- ¼ tsp. chili flakes (optional)
- ¼ tsp. pepper (optional)

Instructions

- Melt some butter in a pan and fry the bacon till it becomes crispy. Remove the bacon from pan and let it cool down.
- Crumble the crispy bacon and place them in a medium bowl.
- Pour the grease left over from the bacon fry into a large bowl and add the remaining ingredients. Mix them well.
- Place the big bowl in the refrigerator for about 15 minutes.
- Take out the cool mixture and make balls of walnut size.
- Roll them over the bacon fry and serve.

52. Delicious Caprese Salad

A quick and simple snack that can easily be altered and turned into dinner

Ingredients (2 servings)

- 1/4 Cup chopped Fresh Basil
- 1 Fresh Tomato
- Fresh Cracked Black Pepper
- 6 Oz. Fresh Mozzarella Cheese
- 3 tbsp. Olive Oil
- Kosher Salt

Instructions

- Make a basil paste by pulsing the chopped basil leaves with 2 tablespoons of olive oil in a food processor.
- Slice the tomato such that you can make out at least 6 slices from the tomato.
- Take Mozzarella cheese and cut slices too.
- Arrange the salad by layering tomato, basil paste, and mozzarella.
- Season the salad with pepper, salt, and extra virgin olive oil.

53. Green Bean Fries

Easy and healthy keto snacks to enjoy with friends and family.

Ingredients (4 servings)

- 1 large egg
- 12 oz. green beans
- 2/3 cup grated parmesan
- 1/4 tsp. black pepper
- 1/2 tsp. pink Himalayan salt
- 1/4 tsp. paprika (optional)
- 1/2 tsp. garlic powder (optional)

Instructions

- The green beans should be dry and the sides must be snipped.
- Preheat the oven to 400°F
- Take a shallow plate and mix the grated parmesan cheese with seasonings.
- Take a bowl that is large enough to drench the beans. Whisk an egg in the bowl and drench green beans in the beaten eggs.
- Take out the green beans and press them gently over the Parmesan cheese mixture. Also, sprinkle some cheese over the beans. Toss them gently with your hands.
- Take your largest baking sheet and place the green beans on it.
- Bake it for about 10 minutes and keep checking if the cheese has turned a slight golden.
- Once the beans cool down to serve them with ranch dressing.

54. Spicy Party Mix

If you are preparing for kids it is a healthy snack and if you want to enjoy it yourself it's a great side dish with cocktails.

Ingredients (2 servings)

- 1 cup pecans
- 1 cup raw cashews
- 2 tbsp. olive oil
- 1 cup sliced almonds
- 1 tsp. chipotle powder
- 3 tbsp. chili powder
- 1 cup golden raisins
- 1 tsp. Celtic sea salt

Instructions

- Take a large bowl and put the nuts in it. Toss it with oil.
- Sprinkle chipotle, chili and salt over the nuts. Keep tossing so that they incorporate.
- Spread the mixture on a large cookie sheet and bake at 350° for about 8 to 10minutes.
- Remove it from the oven and let it cool down. Once cooled toss the raisins in.

55. Herb Stuffed Mushrooms

This recipe may be a veggie one but it is low carb and perfect for snacks.

Ingredients (4 servings)

- 1 pound white button mushrooms
- ¼ cup minced parsley
- 8 ounces' goat cheese
- 1 tsp. minced garlic
- 1 Tbsp. minced chives
- ¼ tsp. Celtic sea salt

Instructions

- Take a paper towel and wipe the mushrooms gently.
- After removing the stems place the mushrooms on a baking sheet lined with parchment paper.
- Place goat cheese, chives, parsley, garlic, and salt in a food processor
- Process it till everything gets blended nicely.
- Scoop a teaspoon into the mushroom.
- Bake the mushrooms at 350°F for about 20 to 25 minutes. You can understand it's done when the goat cheese mixture with turn slightly brown.
- It is now ready to serve.

Chapter 4.5

Keto Desserts recipes

Here is a collection of some delicious desserts that will not only help you maintain your Ketogenic diet but also make every occasion special.

56. Creamsicles

By using fresh orange juice for making this creamsicle you get a tangy taste that is sweet too!

Ingredients (8 servings)

- 1 can full-fat coconut milk
- ½ cup freshly squeezed orange juice
- ½ tsp. vanilla stevia
- ¼ cup lemon juice
- 1 Tbsp. sunflower lecithin powder
- 1½ tsp. orange extract

Instructions

- Blend orange juice, coconut milk and lemon juice in a blender.
- Similarly blend stevia, orange extract, and lecithin until smooth.
- Take Popsicle molds and pour in the mixture.
- Put them in the freezer and set time of 30 minutes.
- After 30minutes, remove the semi-frozen popsicles from freezer and place sticks in them.
- Freeze for 3 hours and Serve

57. Mojito Popsicles

Give your taste buds the feelings of lime dipped in mint sauce.

Ingredients (8 servings)

- 2 cups water
- ¼ tsp. stevia
- ½ cup lime juice
- 20 mint leaves

Instructions

- Take one quart Mason jar and stir together lime juice, water, and stevia.
- Cut the mints into ribbons.
- Pour the mixture into Popsicle molds.
- Add the mint ribbon in all the popsicles.
- Put them in the freezer and set time of 30 minutes.
- After 30minutes, remove the semi-frozen popsicles from freezer and place sticks in them.
- Freeze for 3 hours and Serve

58. Keto Brownies

Brownies are always favorite and when they are low carb nothing like that.

Ingredients (8 servings)

- 1 cup macadamia nuts
- 3 large eggs
- ¼ tsp. baking soda
- ¼ tsp. Celtic sea salt
- 3 ounces chopped 100% dark chocolate
- 2 tbsp. erythritol
- ½ cup melted coconut oil
- 1 tsp. vanilla stevia

Instructions

- Pulse macadamia nuts, baking soda, and salt in a food processor until you get the texture of gravel.
- Pulse in coconut oil and chocolate until smooth
- Pulse in eggs, erythritol, and stevia
- Transfer this mixture to 8x8 baking dish.
- Put it in the oven and bake for 22-25 minutes at 350°F.
- Cool it for one hour and serve.

59. 2-Ingredient Chocolate Pudding

Yes, prepare this tasty chocolate pudding with only two ingredients.

Ingredients (6 servings)

- 1 cup chocolate chips
- 1 can full-fat coconut milk

Instructions

- Mix coconut milk and chocolate in a saucepan and heat it over a low flame.
- Keep it stirring constantly so that the chocolate is melted.
- Take six ½ cup mason jars and divide the mixture in them.
- Refrigerate the mixture for about 3 hours.
- Take out and serve.

60. Chocolate Chia Pudding

Ingredients (4 servings)

- 1 can blend full fat coconut milk
- 1 cup water
- 2 Tbsp. cacao powder
- ¼ cup chia seeds
- ⅛ tsp. Celtic sea salt
- ⅛ tsp. vanilla stevia

Instructions

- Take one-quart mason jar and combine blended coconut milk, chia seeds, and water in it. Shake it well.
- Then add stevia, cacao powder, and salt and shake again.
- Refrigerate it overnight so that the chia seeds absorb the liquid and get softer.
- It is ready to serve the next day.

61. Crunchy Keto Berry Mousse

This crunchy keto mousse is so simple that any cook can place it at the dinner table with little effort.

Ingredients (4 servings)

- 1 cup heavy whipping cream
- 7/8 oz. chopped pecan nuts
- 12/3 oz. mixed berries frozen or fresh
- 1/8 tsp. vanilla extract
- ¼ lemon the zest

Instructions

- In a bowl pour cream and whip it with a hand mixer so that a soft peak is formed.
- Add vanilla and lemon zest towards the end.
- Add nuts and berries to the whipped cream. Constantly keep it stirring.
- Cover the bowl with plastic wrap and place it in the refrigerator for 3 or more hours.

62. Saffron Pannacotta

A bright yellow and delicious keto finale to end your holiday parties.

Ingredients (4 servings)

- 1⁄3 Tbsp. unflavored powdered gelatin
- 11⁄3 cups heavy whipping cream
- 2⁄3 pinch saffron
- water
- 1⁄6 tsp. vanilla extract
- 2⁄3 Tbsp. chopped almonds (optional)
- 2⁄3 Tbsp. honey (optional)

Instructions

- Take gelatin and mix it with a small amount of water. It is better to follow the instruction of the brand you are using. Keep it aside so that it can bloom.
- Add cream, saffron, vanilla and honey (if you wish) in a saucepan and lower the heat so that the mixture can simmer for few minutes.
- After removing the pan from the stove top add some gelatin. Stir it till the gelatin gets dissolved.
- Pour the mixture into 4 glasses and cover them with plastic wrap. Place the glasses in the refrigerator for about 2 hours.
- Take the almonds and toast it dry in a hot frying pan. Add it at the top of pannacotta along with berries and serve.

63. Cinnamon Coffee Cake

Ingredients (8 servings)

Cake

- 3 large eggs
- 2½ cups almond flour, blanched
- ½ tsp. baking soda
- ¼ tsp. Celtic sea salt
- ½ cup honey
- ¼ cup coconut oil

Topping

- ¼ cup melted coconut oil
- 2 tbsp. ground cinnamon
- ¼ cup coconut sugar
- ½ cup sliced almonds

Instructions

- Take a 9 inch round cake pan and grease it with coconut oil and for dusting it use almond flour.
- Combine almond flour, baking soda, and salt in a food processor.
- Pulse in coconut oil, eggs, and honey.
- Spread the batter made into the greased baking dish.
- To make the topping take a small bowl and combine cinnamon, coconut sugar, coconut oil, and sliced almonds.
- Sprinkle the topping over the batter.
- Bake at 350° for 25-35 minutes
- Cool it and serve

64. Cinnamon Blondie Pecan Bars

Ingredients (8 servings)

The Bars

- 3 large eggs
- 1 cup erythritol
- 6 tbsp. melted unsalted butter
- 2 tsp. s vanilla extract
- 1 Tbsp. cinnamon
- 1 ½ cups almond flour
- 1 tsp. baking powder
- ¼ tsp. s salt

Pecan Glaze

- 2 tbsp. unsalted butter
- 2 tbsp. erythritol
- ¼ cup heavy whipping cream
- 1 cup chopped pecans

Instructions

- Preheat oven to 350°F.
- Take a large mixing bowl and mix 6 tablespoons of melted butter with a cup of erythritol.
- In the same bowl blend the vanilla extract and eggs till it becomes smooth. Set it aside.
- Take another bowl and mix the cinnamon, almond flour, salt and baking powder. Blend it nicely.
- Now add the dry ingredients to the wet ingredients and use a blender to make a smooth mix.
- Grease an 8x8 baking pan and add the batter in it. Set it aside.
- In a small frying pan melt about to tablespoon of unsalted butter till it becomes slightly brown.
- Whisk two tablespoons of erythritol along with heavy whipping cream so that it becomes thick. It will be used as caramel flavor that will be mixed with the pecans.
- Put the baking pan inside the oven, when it starts bubbling add the chopped pecans into it. Mix it for about 3 to 5 minutes.
- Bake the mixture at 350°F for about 20 to 25 minute. You can also check by the look of the pecans. When they seem to be dry it's almost ready.

65. Apple Fritters

Ingredients (8 servings)

- ¼ cup arrowroot powder
- ¼ cup coconut flour
- 3 whisked large eggs
- ¼ tsp. Celtic sea salt
- ¼ cup maple syrup
- 1 peeled and cored apple,
- olive oil for frying

Instructions

- Take a medium bowl and put in arrowroot, coconut flour and salt to combine.
- Mix in maple syrup and the eggs.
- Cut the apple in rings and dip them in the batter.
- Heat oil in a frying pan and put the dipped apple rings in the pan.
- Transfer to paper towel to remove the extra oil.
- Serve it with cinnamon sugar and ice cream.

66. Almond Pulp Macaroons

Ingredients (16 pieces)

- ½ cup dates (remove pits)
- ¼ tsp. Celtic sea salt
- 1 cup almond pulp
- ½ cup shredded unsweetened coconut
- ¼ cup coconut oil

Instructions

- Pulse almond pulp and dates in a food processor till the mixture is smooth.
- Pulse in coconut oil, salt, and shredded coconut
- Take a baking sheet and scoop batter on it.
- Bake at 350°F for about 30 minutes. It should get golden around the edges.
- Cool it down and serve.

67. Strawberry Crisp

Ingredients

- 1 pound sliced strawberries,
- ½ cup blanched almond flour
- 1 Tbsp. palm shortening or butter
- ¼ tsp. Celtic sea salt
- ½ cup blanched slivered almonds

Instructions

- Pile the sliced strawberries in a ramekin and place them on baking sheets.
- Bake strawberries for 30 minutes at 350° F.
- While it is baking make the topping in a food processor.
- Pulse almond flour, butter, and salt until dough form
- Pulse in the slivered almonds briefly
- Remove ramekins from oven when it is done.
- Spoon topping made over baked strawberries
- Bake it again for 20-30 minutes at 350°F, the topping will turn golden-brown
- Remove from oven and serve

68. Raspberry Thumbprint Cookies

Ingredients

- 2 cups blanched almond flour
- ¼ tsp. baking soda
- ¼ tsp. Celtic sea salt
- 2 tbsp. honey
- 3 tbsp. coconut oil
- ¼ cup jam

Instructions

- Combine almond flour, baking soda, and salt in a food processor.
- Pulse in honey and coconut oil until the dough is formed.
- Take a baking sheet that is lined with parchment paper. Scoop the batter on the parchment paper.
- To make an indentation in the middle of the cookies press your thumb in its center.
- Put some jam in the center of each cookie.
- Bake for 8-10 minutes at 350°F until golden brown.
- Let them cool down on the baking sheets and serve.

69. Keto Pumpkin Pie

Ingredients

- 15 oz. canned pumpkin puree
- ½ cup full fat coconut milk
- 3 large eggs
- 1 Tbsp. ground cinnamon
- ½ cup honey
- ⅛ Tsp. Celtic sea salt
- 1 tsp. ground nutmeg
- 1 Keto Pie Crust, unbaked

Instructions

- Combine pumpkin puree and eggs in a food processor.
- Pulse in coconut milk, cinnamon, nutmeg, honey, and salt
- Take a keto pie crust and pour the filling.
- Bake it at 350°F for about 40minutes.
- Let it get cool by storing it in a refrigerator for about 2 hours.

70. Low-Carb Buttercream

Ingredients (4 servings)

- ½ lb. butter, at room temperature
- 1 – 2 tsp. tamari soy sauce
- 2 tsp. s vanilla extract
- 1 – 2 tsp. honey (optional)

Instructions

- To get the distinct praline flavor you need to brown the butter in a saucepan. Remember it must be amber in color and should not get burnt. Combine this butter to soy sauce and you will get the praline flavor.
- Pour the browned butter into a pan and whisk the rest of butter into it gradually. You can use a hand blender to make it fluffy.
- Add any flavor of your choice and if you wish to add honey. It is ready to serve.

Chapter 4.6

Keto Side item recipes

When you are serving lunch or dinner these side items will be perfect mate with your main course. Cook them light and enjoy tight.

71. Keto Mushroom Wild Rice Pilaf

A Mexican recipe that can be served as side dish.

Ingredients (4 servings)

- 1 cup Hemp Seeds
- 3 medium Mushrooms
- 1/2 cup Chicken Broth
- 2 tbsp. Butter
- 1/4 cup Sliced Almonds
- 1/4 tsp. Dried Parsley
- 1/2 tsp. Garlic Powder
- Salt and Pepper

Instructions

- Heat the pan and put butter on it.
- Slice mushrooms and almonds and put them on the heated pan with butter.
- After mushroom is soft add chicken broth, hemp seeds, and seasoning.
- Mix it well by stirring continuously.
- Once it is consistent pour and serve.

72. Keto Creamed Spinach

Spinach is fibrous and the cream added to it makes it's a perfect keto dish.

Ingredients (3 servings)

- 10 oz. Frozen Spinach
- 3 oz. Cream Cheese
- 1/4 tsp. Garlic Powder
- 3 tbsp. Parmesan Cheese
- 1/4 tsp. Onion Powder
- 2 tbsp. Sour Cream
- Salt and Pepper

Instructions

- Use the microwave to defrost the spinach. Add the spinach to a pan on medium heat to boil off the excess water.
- Gradually add cream cheese and seasoning to the pan. Keep stirring till the cream cheese melts down.
- Add parmesan and sour cream and mix them till the spinach is thickened.
- Defrost frozen spinach in the microwave. Add to pan on medium-high heat and let the excess water boil off.

73. Creamy Keto Cauliflower

A perfect side dish of cauliflower to be served with any food.

Ingredients (3 servings)

- 10 oz. riced Cauliflower
- 3 tbsp. Heavy Whipping Cream
- 4 tbsp. Parmesan Cheese
- 1/4 cup Sour Cream
- 2 tbsp. chopped Chives
- 3 tbsp. Butter
- 1/4 tsp. Garlic Powder
- Salt and Pepper

Instructions

- Use a food processor to rice the cauliflower.
- Cover the cauliflower with a paper towel and microwave it for about 5 minutes.
- Add in all other ingredients to the microwaved cauliflower. You may use a blender to make a smooth paste of the ingredients.
- Add chopped chives to the mixture and serve after mixing well.

74. Keto Tater Tots

This is low carb keto side dish.

Ingredients (4 servings with about 8 pieces per serving)

- 1 medium Cauliflower
- 1 large Egg
- ¼ cup grated Parmesan Cheese
- 2 oz. shredded Mozzarella Cheese,
- ½ tsp. Garlic Powder
- ½ tsp. Onion Powder
- 2 tsp. Psyllium Husk Powder
- 1 cup Frying Oil
- Salt and Pepper to Taste

Instructions

- Cut the cauliflower florets and steam them till they are tender.
- Pulse them in a food processor till they resemble like mashed potatoes. Wring away the excess water.
- Add egg, cheese, and spices to cauliflower. Mix it gently till the mixture gets thickened.
- At times, you can add psyllium husk powder if required.
- Roll the better into tater tots.
- Deep fry the tater tots till they are brown on each side.
- Cool and serve.

75. Keto Broccoli and Cheese Fritters

This keto side dish is perfect to serve with any Italian dishes.

Ingredients (4 servings with 4 pieces per servings)

The Fritters

- 2 large Eggs
- 3/4 cup Almond Flour
- 4 oz. Fresh Broccoli
- ¼ cup + 3 tbsp. Flaxseed Meal
- 4 oz. Mozzarella Cheese
- Salt and Pepper
- 2 tsp. Baking Powder

The Sauce

- ¼ cup Mayonnaise
- ½ tbsp. Lemon Juice
- ¼ cup Fresh Chopped Dill
- Salt and Pepper

Instructions

- Put broccoli in the food processor and process it till it is completely broken down.
- Mix the other dry ingredients together with the broccoli.
- Add egg to the mixture and mix it again.
- Roll out balls out of the batter and coat the balls with flaxseed meal.
- Heat the deep fryer and fry the fritters till they are golden brown.
- Take the ingredients for sauce in a mixing bowl and mix them to make the dip.
- Serve the fried fritters with the zesty dip.

76. Keto Begedil Potato Patties

It's different and will surely make your taste buds feel the difference.

Ingredients (3 servings)

- 3.5 oz. Cauliflower
- 3.5 oz. Rutabaga
- 4 tbsp. Ground Beef
- 2 small Shallots
- 1 tbsp. chopped Green Onion
- 1 tbsp. chopped Celery Leaves
- 1 large Egg (only little is used)
- ½ tsp. Pepper (White or Black)
- ¼tsp. Salt
- 4 tbsp. Coconut Oil

Instructions

- Slice the rutabaga and cut the cauliflower.
- Fry the rutabaga in coconut oil until it turns brown.
- Cook the cauliflower till they are soft.
- Pound both in a food processor.
- Fry the sliced shallots in coconut oil till they turn crispy and brown.
- Sauté the ground beef, if required you can season it with salt and pepper.
- Mix everything in a mixing bowl except the eggs.
- Make small patties of the mixture and coat them with egg solution.
- Fry the patties in batches and serve hot.

77. Zesty Shrimp in Garlic Sauce

You can serve them as a side dish or enjoy them as snacks too.

Ingredients (2 servings)

- ½ lb. large shrimp
- 3 cloves garlic
- ¼ cup olive oil
- 1 wedge lemon
- ¼ tsp. cayenne
- Salt and pepper

Instructions

- Take a small pan and pour olive oil in it. Add cayenne and minced garlic.
- Cook the garlic on low heat till it leaves fragrant.
- Devein the shrimps after peeling them and cook them on both sides for few minutes.
- Season it with pepper and salt.
- Before serving squeeze the lemon wedge on the shrimp.

78. Tzimmes

A perfect Jewish side dish that can garner your dining table nicely.

Ingredients (6 servings)

- 2 pounds' carrots
- ½ cup dried apricots
- ½ cup prunes
- 2 cups orange juice, freshly squeezed
- ¼ tsp. Celtic sea salt
- 1 tsp. ground cinnamon

Instructions

- Place carrots (cut into ½-inch pieces), apricots (cut in half), prunes (cut in half), and orange juice in a baking dish
- Sprinkle with salt and cinnamon
- Cover the dish
- Put it in the oven and Bake at 350°F for 60-80 minutes

79. Simple Braised Greens

Enjoy these greens with any food item as a side dish.

Ingredients (single serving)

- 1 Tbsp. olive oil
- 4 ounces mixed greens (collard, kale, mustard, or any other greens of your choice)
- ⅛ tsp. Celtic sea salt
- 1 clove garlic, minced
- ¼ tsp. red pepper flakes

Instructions

- Chop the greens and keep them aside.
- Take a large skillet and heat oil in it
- Add the greens and stir it to coat it with oil
- Add salt, garlic and pepper when the greens are wilted.
- Keep stirring till the greens become tender.

80. Mediterranean Portobello Slices

A simple side dish that makes continental food items more interesting.

Ingredients (4 servings)

- 12 oz. Portobello mushroom
- 2 tbsp. olive oil
- 1/2 tsp. tarragon
- 2 tbsp. balsamic vinegar
- 1/2 tsp. basil
- 1/2 tsp. rosemary
- 1/2 tsp. thyme
- pink Himalayan sea salt

Instructions

- The mushroom should be sliced in 1/2" thick.
- After heating the grill whisk balsamic vinegar, herbs and olive oil together.
- Take the mixture of vinegar and brush it on both sides of the sliced mushrooms.
- Lay the slices on the grill and cook both sides for about 4 to 6 minutes
- Once done sprinkle some pink sea salt and serve.

81. Keto Pumpkin Bread

Serve it as a side dish or use it to make any other item.

Ingredients (6 servings)

- 1 cup blanched almond flour
- 3 large eggs
- 1 Tbsp. pumpkin pie spice
- ¼ tsp. Celtic sea salt
- 2 tbsp. honey
- ½ cup roasted pumpkin
- ½ tsp. baking soda
- ¼ tsp. stevia

Instructions

- Combine almond flour, pumpkin pie spice, baking soda and salt in a food processor.
- Add pumpkin, stevia, honey, and eggs and pulse the mixture for another 2 minutes.
- Take a greased mini loaf pan and pour batter in it.
- Bake at 350°F for 35-45 minutes
- Cool for about 1 hour before serving.

82. Delicious Keto Coleslaw

A perfect side dish to compliment any dish that you serve.

Ingredients (2 servings)

- ¼ Head Savoy Cabbage
- 1 Tbsp. Lemon Juice
- 1/3 Cup Mayonnaise
- 1 tsp. Dijon Mustard
- ¼tsp. Onion Powder
- ¼tsp. Garlic Powder
- 1/8 tsp. Paprika
- ¼tsp. Pepper
- Salt

Instructions

- Chop the savoy cabbage clean in such way that each strand come off from the cabbage cleanly.
- Mix all the other ingredients and add some salt to taste.
- It is ready to be served with any other dish.

83. Nut-Free Cranberry Bread

Serve it with some cranberry sauce and enjoy its taste.

Ingredients

- 5 large eggs
- 1 cup frozen cranberries
- ½ cup coconut flour
- ¼ tsp. Celtic sea salt
- ½ tsp. baking soda
- ½ cup maple syrup
- ½ cup coconut oil

Instructions

- Pulse together coconut flour, baking soda, and salt in a food processor
- Pulse in coconut oil, eggs, and maple syrup
- After removing blades from the food processor add and stir cranberries.
- Pour the batter made into mini loaf pans. They must be greased.
- Bake at 350°F for 35-40 minutes
- Cool it and its ready to serve.

84. Bacon Jammin' Green Beans

Healthy beans in a Keto way to add in the required fat in your diet.

Ingredients (3 servings)

- 2½ Cups Fresh Green Beans
- 1 Tbsp. Olive Oil
- 3 Tbsp. Bacon Jam

Instructions

- Boil water and put in green beans.
- Drain the green beans after boiling for 3 to 4 minutes.
- Put the boiled beans in an ice bath for 2 to 3 minutes.
- Take a pan and sizzle bacon jam and olive oil.
- Dry the green beans and put them in the pan.
- Stir the ingredients and cook for 1 to 2 minutes before serving.

85. Fried Queso Fresco

If you need a lot of fat have these squares. They are best to be served as a side item and fun to enjoy.

Ingredients (4 servings)

- 1 lb. Queso Fresco
- ½ Tbsp. Olive Oil
- 1 Tbsp. Coconut Oil

Instructions

- Cut the cheese into thin rectangles or cubes.
- Heat ½ Tbsp. of olive oil and 1 Tbsp. of coconut oil in a pan.
- After the smoke hits add the cheese and cook until brown on both sides.
- After removing from pan use paper towel to drain the excess grease.

Chapter 4.7

Keto Condiments recipes

While cooking condiments add the right flavor to your food. Hence, if you do not have the perfect flavor of your condiments you cannot enjoy the right taste. Here are certain condiments that will help you get the impeccable flavor from all your cooking.

86. Ranch Dip

This is a simple low carb dressing that goes well with grilled foods, salads, and any other low carb snacks.

Ingredients

- ½ tsp. dried tarragon or dried chives
- ½ tsp. dried dill
- ½ tsp. dried parsley
- ¼ tsp. onion powder
- ¼ tsp. garlic powder
- ⅛ tsp. ground black pepper
- ¼ tsp. sea salt
- Sour cream

Instructions

- Add all ingredients in a bowl and mix it well.
- Put it in the fridge and let it sit for 15 minutes so that the flavors develop.
- In order to dilute it, you can add water or buttermilk.
- Serve as dressing for salads or as a dip.

87. Cranberry Cherry Sauce

A perfect sauce to enrich the taste of your toasts, bread, waffles and pancakes.

Ingredients

- 8 ounce fresh cranberries
- 10-ounce frozen cherries
- 10 drops stevia
- 1 cup freshly squeezed orange juice

Instructions

- Place all the ingredients in a saucepan.
- Bring them to boil and reduce heat.
- Simmer the solution for about 20 minutes. The berries will burst and the sauce will start to thicken.
- Transfer it to a bowl and ready to serve.

88. Herb Butter

Another butter condiment that is low carb and goes well with almost anything.

Ingredients

- 1⁄3 lb. butter
- ½ Tbsp. garlic powder
- 1 garlic clove
- 1 tsp. lemon juice
- 4 tbsp. fresh parsley, chopped
- ½ tsp. salt

Instructions

- Take a small bowl and mix all ingredients thoroughly.
- Keep it in the fridge and serve after 30 minutes.

89. Low-Carb Chocolate and Hazelnut Spread

Spread some hazelnut butter on low carb waffles or pancakes and enjoy.

Ingredients

- 3½ oz. hazelnuts
- 2⁄3 oz. butter
- 2¼ tbsp. coconut oil
- 2⁄3 tsp. vanilla extract
- 2 - 4 tsp. s cocoa powder

Instructions

- Take a frying pan and roast the hazelnuts till they are roasted. Cool it down.
- Take out the shell by placing them on a kitchen towel and rubbing them.
- Pour all ingredients into a blender and make a smooth paste.

90. Hollandaise Sauce

This sauce is extremely low carb hence best keto condiment.

Ingredients

- 4 egg yolks
- 8¾ – 11 oz. butter
- 3 tbsp. lemon juice
- Salt and pepper

Instructions

- You need to use only the egg yolks for this condiment. Place the yolks in some heat resistance bowl.
- Take a pan and melt butter in it.
- Take the melted butter and then slowly beat the butter drop by drop to the egg yolks and keep whisking.
- As the sauce thickens increase the pace. Continue till you have added the whole butter.
- Add lemon juice to taste and salt and pepper too. Need to serve immediately.

91. Orange Ginger Sauce

This sauce goes well with any fries or can even be served with choices of bread.

Ingredients

- ¼ cup olive oil
- 1 Tbsp. honey or agave nectar
- 1 Tbsp. plum vinegar
- 1 Tbsp. freshly grated ginger
- ¼ cup freshly squeezed orange juice,

Instructions

- Take a mason jar and pour in all ingredients
- Shake the jar vigorously so to combine.
- Serve with fries.

92. Mild Curry Seasoning

An Asian curry seasoning that goes well with fish, poultry, vegetarian dishes and sauces too.

Ingredients

- 2 tbsp. ground coriander seeds
- 2 tbsp. ground cumin
- 2 tbsp. turmeric
- ½ Tbsp. ground ginger
- ½ Tbsp. chili flakes
- ½ Tbsp. mustard seeds
- 1 Tbsp. sea salt (optional)

Instructions

- Grind all the ingredients separately.
- Mix all the spices together and pour in a tight lid jar.
- Store the spices in dark and warm place. You can store and use them for 4 to 6 months.

93. Marcon Almond Mayonnaise

Another flavor of mayo to bring variation to your taste buds. Serve it with sandwiches and fries.

Ingredients

- 1 Tbsp. agave nectar
- ¼ cup apple cider vinegar
- ½ cup olive oil
- 2-4 tbsp. macron almonds

Instructions

- Make a puree of agave and vinegar in a blender.
- While the puree is in making drizzle some olive oil so that emulsion is created.
- Even if it does not get emulsified, the almonds will do the thickening.
- Keep adding Tbsp. of almonds till the mixture becomes thick and creamy.

94. Parmesan Butter

This condiment is simple yet it goes well with any meal.

Ingredients

- ⅓ lb. butter
- ¼ tsp. grounded black pepper
- ½ tsp. salt
- 2 oz. grated parmesan cheese

Instructions

- Take butter at room temperature.
- Mix the ingredients in a small bowl and keep it inside the fridge.
- Serve it with chicken, fish or vegetable and let it enrich the taste.

95. Flavored Olive Oil

Bring some change in your cooking with different flavored olive oil.

Ingredients

- Olive oil
- The flavoring of your choice like lemon, herbs, garlic etc.

Instructions

- Take any flavoring item that you wish to add to olive oil.
- Wash them carefully and cut into small pieces as you like.
- Put them in a jar and pour olive oil into it.
- Use when required.

96. Wasabi Mayonnaise

Add fat to your Asian cooking with the help of this delicious mayo. It goes great with chicken or even tuna.

Ingredients

- ½ Tbsp. wasabi paste
- 1 cup mayonnaise

Instructions

- Mix the mayonnaises with the wasabi paste and its ready to serve.

Tips: in order to control the heat and taste start with mixing in little amounts. You can store it in the refrigerator for 4 to 5 days.

97. Italian Seasoning

Italian seasoning is all about the perfect blend of different herbs.

Ingredients

- 1 tsp. dried sage
- 3 tbsp. basil, dried
- 3 tbsp. parsley, dried
- 3 tbsp. dried oregano
- 1 tsp. onion powder
- 1 tsp. dried thyme
- 1 Tbsp. garlic powder
- 1 tsp. dried rosemary
- ¼ tsp. chili flakes
- ¼ tsp. s grounded black pepper
- 1 Tbsp. sea salt (optional)

Instructions

- Grind all the ingredients separately.
- Mix all the spices together and pour in a tight lid jar.
- Store the spices in dark and warm place. You can store and use them for 4 to 6 months.

98. Low-Carb Caesar Dressing

This is a common flavorful dressing that goes well with almost every seafood or chicken item.

Ingredients

- ½ cup grated parmesan cheese
- 1 Tbsp. Dijon mustard
- ½ garlic clove, grated
- 1 pinch grounded black pepper
- ½ cup olive oil
- 1 tsp. red wine vinegar
- 3 – 5 anchovies
- ½ tsp. salt
- ½ lemon, juice it

Instructions

- Take all the ingredients, except salt, in a blender and blend or whisk till it is smooth.
- Add salt to taste and serve

99. Pink Herb Butter

This flavored butter is an item that goes almost with anything.

Ingredients

- 4¾ oz. butter
- ½ garlic clove
- 2 oz. grated parmesan cheese
- 1 Tbsp. coarsely grounded rose pepper
- ¼ tsp. salt
- ½ tsp. white wine vinegar or lime juice

Instructions

- Use the butter at room temperature.
- Add all the ingredients and mix nicely with a hand mixer.
- Ready to serve

100. Homemade Tomato Sauce

This sauce is ideal to serve with fries and use in different cooking.

Ingredients

- 1 1/2 Cups Jarred Tomato Sauce
- 1 Green Bell Pepper
- 1/4 Cup Red Wine
- 1 Tbsp. Butter
- 1 Tbsp. Chopped Thyme

Instructions

- Chop the bell peppers and sauté in butter.
- Add the tomato sauce to it and stir it for 4-5 minutes till it reduces.
- Gradually add red wine, thyme, and mix them well.
- Keep stirring on medium-low heat for about 10 minutes and serve.

This recipe is to cool you down whenever you want

101. Strawberry Lemonade

Ingredients (6 servings)

- 2 cups ice
- 8 cups water
- 6 lemons, juiced
- 1 pint sliced strawberries
- ½ tsp. stevia

Instructions

- Take a large pitcher and pour in ice, water, lemon juice and stevia.
- Add in strawberries and stir. Let the mixture sit for 15 minutes.
- Enjoy cool!

Conclusion

This book is an attempt to help you cook some tasty and mouthwatering ketogenic recipes so that you do not feel odd while you are under Ketogenic diet.

The recipes mentioned here are simple and can be served for different occasions. There is a collection of few traditional dishes too so when you eat them along with your family you will find them astonished.

This book aims to provide you with delicious and easy ketogenic recipes that will help you maintain your diet plan in an interesting way. In a ketogenic diet, you need to cut down the carbs and add in fat. Thus, you'll find that butter is added to many recipes if you need more you can add some more.

Do cook them and enjoy with your family and friend.

Thank you again for downloading this book!

I hope this book could help you to cook delicious Ketogenic recipes.

Finally, if you enjoyed this book, then I'd like to ask you for a favor, would you be kind enough to leave a review for this book on Amazon? It'd be greatly appreciated!

Leave a review for this book on Amazon!

Thank you and good luck!

www.ingramcontent.com/pod-product-compliance
Lightning Source LLC
Chambersburg PA
CBHW020519290526
45786CB00002B/678